THE COMPLETE SJOGREN'S SYNDROME SMOOTHIE COOKBOOK

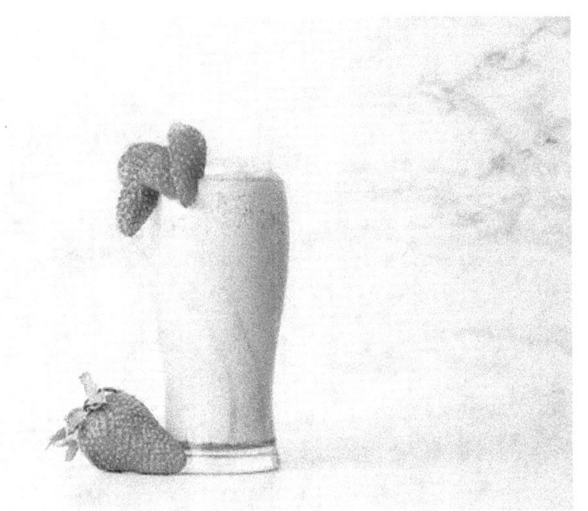

DR. VICKIE STOCK

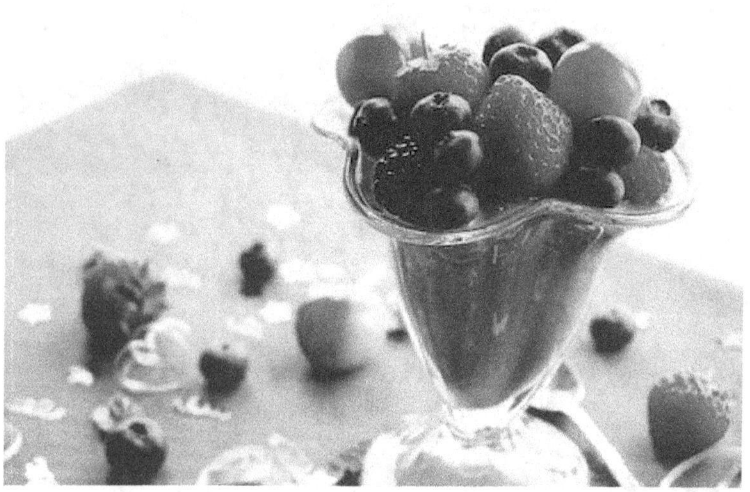

TABLE OF CONTENT

INTRODUCTION TO SJÖGREN'S SYNDROME

Sjögren's Syndrome, named after Swedish ophthalmologist Henrik Sjögren who first identified it in the early 20th century, is a chronic autoimmune disorder that primarily affects the exocrine glands, particularly those responsible for producing tears and saliva.

This syndrome is characterized by a malfunction of the immune system, which mistakenly attacks the body's own moisture-producing glands, leading to symptoms such as dry eyes and dry mouth. While these are the hallmark features, Sjögren's Syndrome can also impact other organs and systems, causing a range of additional complications.

One of the key aspects of Sjögren's Syndrome is its prevalence among women, with a significant majority of patients being female.

The exact cause of the syndrome remains elusive, but both genetic and environmental factors are believed to contribute to its development. The autoimmune nature of Sjögren's Syndrome means that the immune system not only targets the exocrine glands but can also lead to systemic manifestations, affecting joints, skin, and vital organs.

The primary symptoms of Sjögren's Syndrome include persistent dryness of the eyes and mouth, which can result in discomfort, difficulty swallowing, and an increased risk of dental issues. Beyond the hallmark symptoms, individuals with Sjögren's may experience fatigue, joint pain, and various complications related to systemic involvement.

Diagnosis of Sjögren's Syndrome can be challenging, as its symptoms often overlap with those of other autoimmune diseases. A comprehensive evaluation by healthcare professionals, including blood tests and imaging studies, is typically required to confirm the diagnosis.

Managing Sjögren's Syndrome involves a multidisciplinary approach, addressing both the dryness symptoms and potential systemic complications. Treatment may include artificial tears, saliva substitutes, and medications to alleviate systemic manifestations.

Additionally, lifestyle modifications, such as staying hydrated and avoiding environmental triggers, play a crucial role in enhancing the quality of life for individuals living with Sjögren's Syndrome.

As research continues to uncover the complexities of this autoimmune disorder, raising awareness and promoting understanding are essential steps towards improved diagnosis, treatment, and support for those affected by Sjögren's Syndrome.

Definition and Symptoms

Sjögren's Syndrome is a chronic autoimmune disorder characterized by the immune system attacking the body's moisture-producing glands, leading to dryness primarily in the eyes and mouth.

Named after the Swedish ophthalmologist Henrik Sjögren, who first identified the syndrome in the early 20th century, it has since been recognized as a complex condition with various manifestations beyond its initial description.

The defining features of Sjögren's Syndrome are dry eyes and dry mouth, resulting from the immune system's assault on the lacrimal and salivary glands. Patients often experience a persistent sensation of grittiness or irritation in the eyes, and the dryness in the mouth can lead to difficulty swallowing and an increased susceptibility to dental issues.

Beyond the hallmark symptoms, Sjögren's Syndrome can affect multiple organ systems, causing a range of diverse symptoms. Individuals with this syndrome may suffer from fatigue, joint pain, and muscle discomfort, which can significantly impact their quality of life.

Additionally, systemic complications can involve the skin, respiratory system, and various internal organs. The diagnostic process for Sjögren's Syndrome involves a thorough evaluation by healthcare professionals. Blood tests to detect specific antibodies and imaging studies, such as salivary gland scintigraphy, are commonly employed to confirm the diagnosis. It's crucial to note that the symptoms of Sjögren's Syndrome can overlap with those of other autoimmune diseases, making an accurate diagnosis challenging.

As a chronic condition, Sjögren's Syndrome requires ongoing management to address both the dryness symptoms and potential systemic complications. While there is no cure, treatment strategies aim to alleviate discomfort, improve quality of life, and prevent complications.

Increased awareness and understanding of the definition and symptoms of Sjögren's Syndrome are essential for timely diagnosis and appropriate management, empowering individuals affected by this autoimmune disorder to navigate their health journey effectively.

Impact on Daily Life

Sjögren's Syndrome, with its hallmark symptoms of dry eyes and dry mouth, can significantly impact the daily lives of individuals affected by the condition. The pervasive dryness experienced by those with Sjögren's Syndrome extends beyond mere discomfort, influencing various aspects of daily functioning and overall well-being.

One of the most immediate and noticeable impacts is on ocular health. Dry eyes can lead to persistent irritation, a gritty feeling, and increased sensitivity to light. Vision may become blurred, and performing simple tasks such as reading, watching television, or using electronic devices can become challenging. The constant discomfort in the eyes may also affect concentration and productivity, making daily activities more demanding.

The dryness in the mouth, another hallmark of Sjögren's, presents its own set of challenges. Reduced saliva production can result in difficulty swallowing, altered taste sensations, and an increased risk of dental problems such as cavities and gum disease. The overall impact on oral health can affect the enjoyment of meals, leading to dietary adjustments and potential nutritional concerns.

Beyond the eyes and mouth, Sjögren's Syndrome can manifest systemically, contributing to fatigue, joint pain, and muscle discomfort. These symptoms can limit physical activities and may lead to a decreased overall quality of life.

The chronic nature of the condition requires individuals to adapt their daily routines to manage symptoms effectively, often incorporating regular use of artificial tears, lubricating mouth sprays, and other interventions. Moreover, the systemic nature of Sjögren's Syndrome may contribute to a heightened risk of developing complications affecting internal organs.

This aspect necessitates ongoing medical monitoring and management, adding another layer of impact on daily life.

Coping with Sjögren's Syndrome often involves a combination of medical interventions, lifestyle adjustments, and emotional support. Increased awareness of these daily challenges is crucial for fostering understanding and empathy, both within affected communities and among healthcare providers, ultimately contributing to improved management and the enhancement of the daily lives of individuals living with Sjögren's Syndrome.

The Role of Nutrition in Managing Sjögren's Syndrome

The role of nutrition in managing Sjögren's Syndrome is integral to improving the overall well-being of individuals affected by this autoimmune disorder.

While nutrition alone cannot cure the condition, a well-balanced and thoughtful diet can help alleviate symptoms and enhance the quality of life for those living with Sjögren's.

One of the primary challenges faced by individuals with Sjögren's Syndrome is the persistent dryness, particularly in the eyes and mouth. Adequate hydration is crucial to combat these symptoms, and individuals are often advised to increase their water intake.

Sipping water throughout the day helps maintain moisture in the mucous membranes, easing the discomfort associated with dryness.

Incorporating foods rich in omega-3 fatty acids can be beneficial for managing inflammation, a common feature of autoimmune conditions like Sjögren's Syndrome. Fatty fish, flaxseeds, chia seeds, and walnuts are excellent sources of omega-3s and can be included in the diet to support overall health.

Certain vitamins and minerals play a crucial role in immune function and maintaining healthy tissues. Foods high in vitamin A, vitamin C, and zinc can contribute to the overall well-being of individuals with Sjögren's Syndrome.

Vitamin A-rich foods like sweet potatoes and carrots support eye health, while vitamin C from citrus fruits and zinc from nuts and seeds help bolster the immune system.

Anti-inflammatory foods, such as fruits, vegetables, and whole grains, are essential components of a Sjögren's-friendly diet. These foods may help mitigate systemic inflammation and provide a range of nutrients beneficial for overall health.

Considering the potential challenges in chewing and swallowing associated with dry mouth, incorporating smoothies and soft, hydrating foods into the diet can be a practical approach. Smoothies, in particular, offer a convenient way to pack in nutrients, providing hydration and nourishment in an easily digestible form.

While nutritional strategies are not a substitute for medical treatment, they can complement other aspects of Sjögren's Syndrome management.

Consulting with healthcare professionals or registered dietitians can help tailor dietary recommendations to individual needs, ensuring a comprehensive approach to supporting health and well-being in the context of Sjögren's Syndrome.

Nutritional Challenges for Sjögren's Patients

Nutritional challenges for individuals with Sjögren's Syndrome stem from the impact of the condition on the exocrine glands, particularly those responsible for producing saliva and tears.

The persistent dryness experienced by Sjögren's patients can significantly affect their ability to eat, drink, and obtain essential nutrients, presenting a range of challenges that require thoughtful dietary considerations.

Dry mouth, or xerostomia, is a common symptom in Sjögren's Syndrome. The reduced saliva flow can make chewing and swallowing difficult, leading to a potential aversion to certain foods.

This challenge may result in inadequate calorie intake and a heightened risk of malnutrition, emphasizing the importance of addressing the nutritional needs of individuals with Sjögren's.

The lack of saliva also affects the initial stages of digestion, impairing the breakdown of food in the mouth. This can lead to difficulties in extracting nutrients from ingested food, potentially impacting nutrient absorption and overall nutritional status. Insufficient saliva may also contribute to dental problems, increasing the risk of cavities and gum disease.

Dry eyes can pose challenges related to visual and cognitive aspects of eating. The discomfort and blurred vision associated with dry eyes may affect the ability to read labels, prepare meals, or enjoy the visual appeal of food.

Adequate hydration, typically facilitated by saliva, becomes a crucial concern, requiring conscious efforts to maintain fluid balance through increased water intake.

To address these challenges, individuals with Sjögren's Syndrome may need to adopt dietary modifications, such as choosing softer and moist foods, avoiding dry and crunchy textures, and incorporating hydrating foods like fruits and vegetables.

Regular dental check-ups and good oral hygiene practices are also essential components of managing nutritional challenges associated with Sjögren's Syndrome.

Nutritional support from healthcare professionals, including dietitians, can play a vital role in tailoring dietary recommendations to individual needs, ensuring that Sjögren's patients receive the necessary nutrients despite the challenges posed by dryness symptoms.

Awareness of these nutritional challenges is crucial for fostering a holistic approach to the management of Sjögren's Syndrome and improving the overall well-being of those affected by the condition.

Importance of a Balanced Diet

The importance of a balanced diet cannot be overstated, and it holds particular significance for individuals managing conditions such as Sjögren's Syndrome.

A balanced diet provides the body with the necessary nutrients, vitamins, and minerals essential for overall health and well-being. For those with autoimmune disorders like Sjögren's Syndrome, maintaining a balanced diet becomes paramount to support the immune system, manage symptoms, and improve the quality of life.

A balanced diet encompasses a variety of food groups, including fruits, vegetables, whole grains, lean proteins, and dairy or dairy alternatives. Each food group contributes unique nutrients that play crucial roles in bodily functions.

For individuals with Sjögren's Syndrome, the inclusion of anti-inflammatory foods can be particularly beneficial. These may help mitigate systemic inflammation, a common feature of autoimmune conditions.

Adequate hydration is a cornerstone of a balanced diet, and it is especially vital for individuals with Sjögren's Syndrome, given the chronic dryness they experience.

Proper hydration supports overall health, helps maintain mucous membrane moisture, and can alleviate symptoms like dry mouth and dry eyes. Water, herbal teas, and hydrating foods such as fruits and vegetables contribute to fluid intake.

Balanced nutrition also plays a role in supporting oral health, addressing potential challenges like xerostomia (dry mouth) commonly associated with Sjögren's Syndrome. Foods that stimulate saliva production, such as sugar-free gum or hydrating fruits, can aid in maintaining oral moisture and reducing the risk of dental issues.

Moreover, a balanced diet supports energy levels, helping individuals manage the fatigue often associated with autoimmune conditions. Nutrient-dense foods provide a sustained source of energy, aiding in the overall management of symptoms and enhancing daily functioning.

Consulting with healthcare professionals or registered dietitians can help tailor a balanced diet to meet the specific needs of individuals with Sjögren's Syndrome. A personalized approach to nutrition can contribute to improved symptom management, better overall health, and an enhanced quality of life for those navigating the challenges of autoimmune disorders.

Overview of Smoothies as a Nutritional Solution

An overview of smoothies as a nutritional solution reveals their versatility and efficacy, particularly for individuals managing conditions like Sjögren's Syndrome. Smoothies offer a convenient and palatable way to incorporate essential nutrients, address hydration challenges, and enhance overall well-being.

Smoothies are a blend of fruits, vegetables, liquids, and additional nutritional boosts, creating a delicious and easily digestible concoction. For individuals with Sjögren's Syndrome, where dry mouth and difficulty swallowing are common challenges, the smooth texture of these beverages provides a welcomed solution.

The liquid nature of smoothies facilitates hydration, crucial for maintaining mucous membrane moisture and combating the persistent dryness associated with the condition.

One key advantage of smoothies is their adaptability to specific dietary needs. They can be tailored to include anti-inflammatory ingredients, vitamins, and minerals that support immune function and reduce inflammation – important considerations for individuals with autoimmune disorders like Sjögren's Syndrome.

Ingredients such as berries, leafy greens, and omega-3-rich seeds can be seamlessly blended into a smoothie to create a nutrient-dense and anti-inflammatory beverage.

Smoothies also offer a creative platform for incorporating hydrating foods that contribute to overall fluid intake. Ingredients like water-rich fruits (e.g., watermelon, cucumber) and liquid bases such as coconut water or almond milk can enhance the hydrating properties of a smoothie, addressing the dual challenge of dry eyes and dry mouth.

In addition to their nutritional benefits, smoothies can be a practical solution for those with difficulties in chewing or swallowing solid foods. The easily digestible nature of smoothies ensures that essential nutrients are readily absorbed, supporting individuals with Sjögren's Syndrome in maintaining proper nutrition.

As a convenient and customizable nutritional solution, smoothies provide a refreshing way for individuals managing Sjögren's Syndrome to address specific dietary challenges while enjoying a tasty and hydrating beverage.

Integrating smoothies into a well-balanced diet can contribute to improved overall health and assist in the management of symptoms associated with autoimmune conditions.

Benefits of Smoothies for Sjögren's Patients

The benefits of incorporating smoothies into the diet of individuals with Sjögren's Syndrome are multifaceted, offering a range of advantages that address the unique challenges posed by this autoimmune disorder.

Smoothies serve as a valuable nutritional tool, providing hydration, convenience, and tailored nutrient support for those managing the symptoms of Sjögren's.

Hydration: Persistent dryness, particularly in the eyes and mouth, is a hallmark symptom of Sjögren's Syndrome. Smoothies, often made with hydrating ingredients like fruits and liquid bases, contribute significantly to overall fluid intake.

Maintaining adequate hydration is crucial for individuals with Sjögren's, as it helps alleviate symptoms associated with dry mucous membranes.

Nutrient Density: Smoothies offer a concentrated source of essential nutrients in an easily digestible form. Ingredients such as fruits, vegetables, and seeds can be blended together to create a nutrient-dense beverage.

This is particularly beneficial for individuals with Sjögren's Syndrome, as it ensures a comprehensive intake of vitamins, minerals, and antioxidants, supporting overall health and potentially addressing nutritional deficiencies.

Texture Modification: Chewing and swallowing difficulties, often associated with dry mouth, can be alleviated through the consumption of smoothies. The smooth and liquid consistency of these beverages requires minimal effort in terms of mastication, making them an ideal option for those with challenges in oral processing.

Anti-Inflammatory Potential: Tailoring smoothies with anti-inflammatory ingredients, such as berries, leafy greens, and omega-3-rich seeds, can provide an additional layer of support for individuals with autoimmune conditions like Sjögren's Syndrome. These ingredients may help mitigate inflammation, a common feature of autoimmune disorders.

Convenience and Variety: Smoothies offer a convenient and time-efficient way to diversify the diet. They can be easily customized with different ingredients, allowing individuals to experiment with flavors and nutritional profiles, thus preventing dietary monotony.

Incorporating smoothies into the daily routine of individuals with Sjögren's Syndrome can contribute significantly to their overall well-being.

As a palatable and adaptable nutritional solution, smoothies address hydration needs, provide essential nutrients, and offer a practical option for individuals facing challenges related to dryness and oral discomfort.

Key Nutrients for Sjögren's Syndrome

Ensuring an optimal intake of key nutrients is crucial for individuals with Sjögren's Syndrome, an autoimmune disorder characterized by dry eyes and dry mouth. These nutrients play pivotal roles in supporting overall health, managing symptoms, and potentially alleviating the impact of autoimmune conditions on the body.

Here are some key nutrients that individuals with Sjögren's Syndrome should consider incorporating into their diet:

Omega-3 Fatty Acids: Found in fatty fish (such as salmon and mackerel), flaxseeds, chia seeds, and walnuts, omega-3 fatty acids are known for their anti-inflammatory properties. Including these foods in the diet may help manage inflammation, which is often elevated in autoimmune conditions like Sjögren's Syndrome.

Vitamins and Minerals: Ensuring an adequate intake of vitamins and minerals is essential. Vitamin A, found in sweet potatoes and carrots, supports eye health. Vitamin C, abundant in citrus fruits, strawberries, and bell peppers, is vital for immune function and collagen production. Zinc, present in nuts and seeds, contributes to immune health and wound healing.

Calcium and Vitamin D: These nutrients are crucial for bone health, and individuals with Sjögren's Syndrome may be at an increased risk of bone density issues. Dairy products, fortified plant-based milks, leafy greens, and exposure to sunlight are excellent sources of calcium and vitamin D.

Hydration: While not a specific nutrient, maintaining adequate hydration is fundamental for those with Sjögren's Syndrome. Water-rich fruits like watermelon and cucumber, along with herbal teas, contribute to overall fluid intake, helping combat the dryness associated with the condition.

Anti-Inflammatory Foods: In addition to specific nutrients, incorporating anti-inflammatory foods into the diet can be beneficial. Berries, leafy greens, and turmeric are examples of foods with anti-inflammatory properties that may help manage symptoms associated with autoimmune conditions.

Individuals with Sjögren's Syndrome are encouraged to work with healthcare professionals, including registered dietitians, to personalize their dietary approach based on individual needs and preferences. A well-balanced and nutrient-rich diet can contribute to improved overall health and potentially enhance the management of Sjögren's Syndrome symptoms.

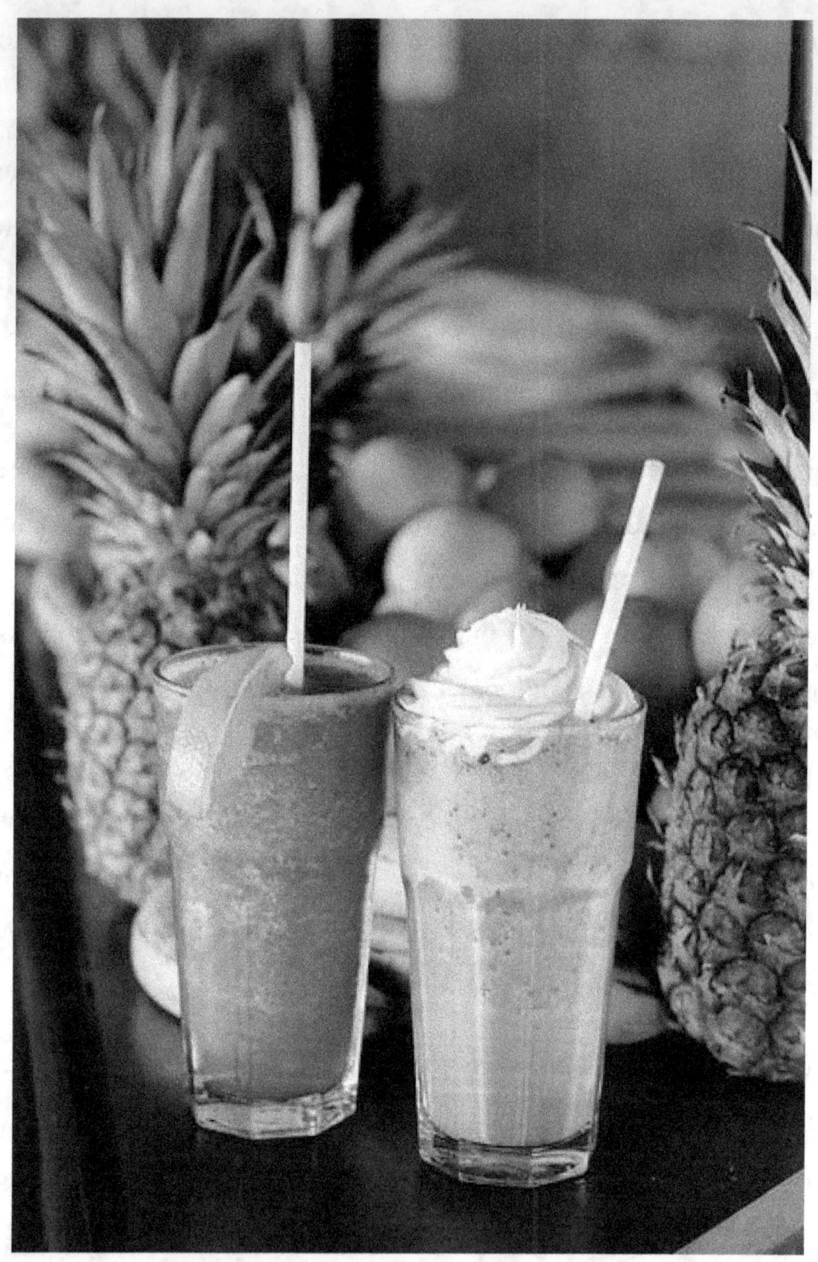

SJOGRE'S SYNDROME SMOOTHIE RECIPES

1. Berry Bliss Smoothie

Ingredients:

- 1 cup mixed berries (blueberries, strawberries, raspberries)
- 1/2 banana
- 1/2 cup Greek yogurt
- 1 tablespoon chia seeds
- 1 cup coconut water
- Ice cubes (optional)

Instructions:

- Combine all ingredients in a blender.
- Blend until smooth.
- Pour into a glass and enjoy!

Benefits:

This antioxidant-rich smoothie provides hydration, immune support, and anti-inflammatory properties, addressing common concerns for Sjögren's Syndrome patients.

2. Green Healing Elixir

Ingredients:

- 1 cup kale leaves (stems removed)
- 1/2 cucumber (peeled)
- 1/2 green apple (cored)
- 1/2 avocado
- 1 tablespoon flaxseeds
- 1 cup coconut water

Instructions:

1. Blend all ingredients until well combined.
2. Adjust thickness with water if needed.
3. Pour into a glass and savor the freshness!

Benefits:

This green smoothie provides a nutrient-packed blend with anti-inflammatory effects, supporting overall health and well-being.

3. Tropical Hydration Delight

- Ingredients:
- 1 cup pineapple chunks
- 1/2 mango (peeled and diced)
- 1/2 banana
- 1/2 cup coconut milk

- 1 tablespoon hemp seeds

- Ice cubes (optional)

Instructions:

- Blend all ingredients until smooth.

- Adjust consistency with additional coconut milk.

- Pour into a tropical glass and enjoy the hydrating flavors!

Benefits:

Rich in vitamins, minerals, and hydration, this tropical smoothie is refreshing and supports immune function.

4. Creamy Almond Berry Blend

Ingredients:

- 1 cup mixed berries (strawberries, blackberries, blueberries)

- 1/2 cup almond butter

- 1/2 cup plain yogurt

- 1 tablespoon honey

- 1 cup almond milk

- Ice cubes (optional)

Instructions:

- Combine all ingredients in a blender.

- Blend until creamy and smooth.

- Pour into a glass and relish the nutty-berry goodness!

Benefits:

This smoothie is rich in antioxidants, healthy fats, and protein, providing sustained energy and immune support.

5. Citrus Burst Revitalizer

Ingredients:

- 1 orange (peeled and segmented)
- 1/2 cup pineapple chunks
- 1/2 lemon (juiced)
- 1 tablespoon chia seeds
- 1 cup coconut water
- Ice cubes (optional)

Instructions:

- Blend all ingredients until citrusy perfection is achieved.
- Adjust thickness with coconut water if needed.
- Pour into a glass and experience the zesty revitalization!

Benefits:

Packed with vitamin C and hydration, this citrus smoothie boosts immune health and refreshes the palate.

6. Spinach Berry Powerhouse

Ingredients:

- 1 cup spinach leaves
- 1/2 cup mixed berries (strawberries, blueberries)
- 1/2 cup pineapple chunks
- 1/2 banana
- 1 tablespoon almond butter
- 1 cup water or coconut water

Instructions:

- Blend all ingredients until the mixture is smooth.
- Adjust consistency with water or coconut water as desired.
- Pour into a glass and enjoy this nutrient-packed green smoothie!

Benefits:

This smoothie combines the power of leafy greens with antioxidant-rich berries, providing vitamins, minerals, and a natural energy boost.

7. Creamy Avocado Citrus Splash

Ingredients:

- 1/2 avocado
- 1/2 cup orange segments

- 1/2 lime (juiced)

- 1 tablespoon chia seeds

- 1/2 cup coconut milk

- Ice cubes (optional)

Instructions:

- Blend all ingredients until creamy and well-combined.

- Adjust thickness with coconut milk or water.

- Pour into a glass and relish the creamy avocado goodness with a citrusy splash!

Benefits:

This smoothie offers a dose of healthy fats from avocado, along with immune-boosting vitamin C from citrus fruits.

8. Turmeric Mango Delight

Ingredients:

- 1 cup mango chunks

- 1/2 teaspoon turmeric powder

- 1/2 teaspoon ginger (grated)

- 1/2 banana

- 1 cup almond milk

- 1 tablespoon honey (optional)

Instructions:

- Blend all ingredients until smooth.
- Adjust sweetness with honey if desired.
- Pour into a glass and savor the tropical turmeric delight!

Benefits:

Turmeric and ginger bring anti-inflammatory properties to this smoothie, complementing the natural sweetness of mango.

9. Blueberry Almond Bliss

Ingredients:

- 1 cup blueberries
- 1/2 cup plain yogurt
- 1/2 cup almond milk
- 1 tablespoon almond flour
- 1 tablespoon flaxseeds
- Ice cubes (optional)

Instructions:

- Blend all ingredients until creamy and well-incorporated.
- Adjust thickness with almond milk.
- Pour into a glass and enjoy the delightful blend of blueberries and almonds!

Benefits:

Rich in antioxidants and healthy fats, this smoothie provides a satisfying and nourishing treat.

10. Coconut Kale Green Refresher

Ingredients:

- 1 cup kale leaves (stems removed)
- 1/2 cup coconut water
- 1/2 cup pineapple chunks
- 1/2 green apple (cored)
- 1 tablespoon coconut flakes
- Ice cubes (optional)

Instructions:

- Blend all ingredients until smooth.
- Adjust thickness with additional coconut water.
- Pour into a glass and experience the tropical green refreshment!

Benefits:

This green smoothie combines the hydrating properties of coconut water with the nutritional punch of kale and pineapple.

11. Raspberry Coconut Dream

Ingredients:

- 1 cup raspberries
- 1/2 cup coconut milk
- 1/2 banana
- 1 tablespoon shredded coconut
- 1 tablespoon hemp seeds
- Ice cubes (optional)

Instructions:

- Blend all ingredients until smooth and creamy.
- Adjust thickness with additional coconut milk.
- Pour into a glass and indulge in the delightful raspberry-coconut combination!

Benefits:

This smoothie combines the antioxidant power of raspberries with the hydrating and nutrient-rich properties of coconut.

12. Minty Melon Cooler

Ingredients:

- 1 cup melon cubes (cantaloupe or honeydew)
- 1/2 cucumber (peeled and sliced)
- 1/4 cup fresh mint leaves

- 1/2 lime (juiced)

- 1 tablespoon chia seeds

- 1 cup water

Instructions:

- Blend all ingredients until smooth.

- Adjust thickness with water if needed.

- Pour into a glass and savor the refreshing minty melon goodness!

Benefits:

This hydrating smoothie provides a cooling effect with the combination of melon, cucumber, and mint, perfect for relieving dryness.

13. Pomegranate Green Tea Elixir

Ingredients:

- 1/2 cup pomegranate seeds

- 1/2 cup brewed green tea (cooled)

- 1/2 banana

- 1 tablespoon honey

- 1/2 teaspoon matcha powder

- Ice cubes (optional)

Instructions:

- Blend all ingredients until well combined.
- Adjust sweetness with honey if needed.
- Pour into a glass and enjoy the antioxidant-rich elixir!

Benefits:

Packed with antioxidants from pomegranate and green tea, this smoothie provides a refreshing and energizing boost.

14. Cherry Almond Protein Boost

Ingredients:

- 1 cup cherries (pitted)
- 1/2 cup almond milk
- 1/2 cup Greek yogurt
- 1 tablespoon almond butter
- 1 tablespoon chia seeds
- Ice cubes (optional)

Instructions:

- Blend all ingredients until smooth and creamy.
- Adjust thickness with additional almond milk.
- Pour into a glass and relish the protein-packed goodness!

Benefits:

This smoothie combines the natural sweetness of cherries with the protein and healthy fats from almond butter and chia seeds.

15. Banana Cocoa Smooth Indulgence

Ingredients:

- 1 banana
- 1 tablespoon cocoa powder
- 1/2 cup plain yogurt
- 1 tablespoon peanut butter
- 1 cup almond milk
- Ice cubes (optional)

Instructions:

- Blend all ingredients until smooth and velvety.
- Adjust thickness with almond milk if desired.
- Pour into a glass and treat yourself to this indulgent yet nutritious smoothie!

Benefits:

Rich in potassium from bananas and antioxidants from cocoa, this smoothie offers a satisfying and guilt-free treat.

16. Mango Turmeric Sunshine

Ingredients:

- 1 cup mango chunks
- 1/2 teaspoon turmeric powder
- 1/2 cup plain yogurt
- 1 tablespoon honey
- 1 cup coconut water
- Ice cubes (optional)

Instructions:

- Blend all ingredients until smooth.
- Adjust sweetness with honey as needed.
- Pour into a glass and bask in the tropical sunshine flavors!

Benefits:

This smoothie combines the tropical sweetness of mango with the anti-inflammatory properties of turmeric.

17. Pineapple Mint Cooler

Ingredients:

- 1 cup pineapple chunks
- 1/4 cup fresh mint leaves
- 1/2 cucumber (peeled and sliced)
- 1/2 lime (juiced)

- 1 tablespoon chia seeds

- 1 cup water

Instructions:

- Blend all ingredients until smooth.

- Adjust thickness with water if required.

- Pour into a glass and relish the refreshing pineapple-mint coolness!

Benefits:

Hydrating and rejuvenating, this smoothie combines the tropical sweetness of pineapple with the cooling effect of mint.

18. Blueberry Oat Powerhouse

Ingredients:

- 1 cup blueberries

- 1/2 cup rolled oats

- 1/2 cup Greek yogurt

- 1 tablespoon almond butter

- 1 cup almond milk

- Ice cubes (optional)

Instructions:

- Blend all ingredients until creamy and well-incorporated.

- Adjust thickness with additional almond milk.

- Pour into a glass and enjoy the nutrient-packed blueberry-oat goodness!

Benefits:

This smoothie provides a hearty mix of antioxidants from blueberries and fiber from oats for sustained energy.

19. Kiwi Citrus Splash

Ingredients:

- 2 kiwis (peeled and sliced)
- 1/2 cup orange segments
- 1/2 lemon (juiced)
- 1 tablespoon honey
- 1 cup coconut water
- Ice cubes (optional)
- Instructions:
- Blend all ingredients until smooth.
- Adjust sweetness with honey as desired.
- Pour into a glass and revel in the zesty kiwi-citrus splash!

Benefits:

Rich in vitamin C, this smoothie provides a refreshing and immune-boosting combination of kiwi and citrus.

20. Peach Basil Bliss

Ingredients:

- 1 cup peach slices (fresh or frozen)
- 1/4 cup fresh basil leaves
- 1/2 banana
- 1 tablespoon chia seeds
- 1 cup almond milk
- Ice cubes (optional)

Instructions:

- Blend all ingredients until smooth.
- Adjust thickness with additional almond milk.
- Pour into a glass and savor the unique peach-basil bliss!

Benefits:

This smoothie offers a delightful blend of sweet peaches with the aromatic freshness of basil, providing antioxidants and hydration.

21. Apple Cinnamon Comfort

Ingredients:

1 apple (cored and sliced)

1/2 teaspoon cinnamon

1/2 cup oats

- 1 tablespoon almond butter

- 1 cup almond milk

- Ice cubes (optional)

Instructions:

- Blend all ingredients until smooth.

- Adjust thickness with almond milk.

- Pour into a glass and relish the comforting combination of apple and cinnamon!

Benefits:

This smoothie provides a heartwarming blend of fiber from oats, antioxidants from apples, and the cozy flavor of cinnamon.

22. Mixed Berry Chia Delight

Ingredients:

- 1 cup mixed berries (strawberries, blueberries, raspberries)

- 2 tablespoons chia seeds

- 1/2 cup Greek yogurt

- 1 tablespoon honey

- 1 cup coconut water

- Ice cubes (optional)

Instructions:

- Blend all ingredients except chia seeds until smooth.

- Stir in chia seeds and let it sit for 5 minutes to thicken.

- Pour into a glass and enjoy the chia-infused berry delight!

Benefits:

Loaded with antioxidants and omega-3 fatty acids from chia seeds, this smoothie supports overall health and hydration.

23. Banana Peanut Butter Protein Punch

Ingredients:

- 1 banana

- 2 tablespoons peanut butter

- 1/2 cup oats

- 1 scoop protein powder (vanilla or chocolate)

- 1 cup almond milk

- Ice cubes (optional)

Instructions:

- Blend all ingredients until creamy and well-incorporated.

- Adjust thickness with almond milk.

- Pour into a glass and relish the protein-packed punch!

Benefits:

This smoothie provides a satisfying combination of protein, healthy fats, and energy-boosting carbs for a nutritious snack or meal replacement.

24. Watermelon Mint Quencher

Ingredients:

- 2 cups watermelon cubes
- 1/4 cup fresh mint leaves
- 1/2 lime (juiced)
- 1 tablespoon chia seeds
- 1 cup coconut water
- Ice cubes (optional)

Instructions:

- Blend watermelon, mint, and lime juice until smooth.
- Stir in chia seeds and let it sit for 5 minutes to thicken.
- Pour into a glass and enjoy the hydrating watermelon-mint quencher!

Benefits:

Refreshing and hydrating, this smoothie combines the natural sweetness of watermelon with the cooling effect of mint.

25. Spinach Pineapple Paradise

Ingredients:

- 1 cup spinach leaves
- 1 cup pineapple chunks
- 1/2 banana

- 1/2 cup coconut milk

- 1 tablespoon hemp seeds

- Ice cubes (optional)

Instructions:

- Blend all ingredients until smooth.

- Adjust thickness with coconut milk.

- Pour into a glass and escape to the spinach-pineapple paradise!

Benefits:

This green smoothie packs a nutrient punch with the goodness of spinach, pineapple, and omega-3-rich hemp seeds.

26. Acai Berry Boost

Ingredients:

- 1 packet frozen acai puree

- 1/2 cup mixed berries (strawberries, blueberries)

- 1/2 banana

- 1 tablespoon almond butter

- 1 cup almond milk

- Ice cubes (optional)

Instructions:

- Blend the acai puree, berries, banana, almond butter, and almond milk until smooth.
- Adjust thickness with additional almond milk.
- Pour into a glass and enjoy the antioxidant-rich acai berry boost!

Benefits:

Acai berries are known for their high antioxidant content, supporting immune health and providing a deliciously rich flavor to this smoothie.

27. Carrot Orange Zinger

Ingredients:

- 1 large carrot (peeled and sliced)
- 1 orange (peeled and segmented)
- 1/2 cup Greek yogurt
- 1 tablespoon honey
- 1 cup water or coconut water
- Ice cubes (optional)

Instructions:

- Blend the carrot, orange segments, Greek yogurt, honey, and water or coconut water until smooth.

- Adjust thickness with additional liquid.
- Pour into a glass and savor the zesty carrot-orange zinger!

Benefits:

This smoothie provides a burst of vitamin C from oranges and beta-carotene from carrots, promoting immune support and vibrant skin health.

28. Mango Basil Refresher

Ingredients:

- 1 cup mango chunks
- 1/4 cup fresh basil leaves
- 1/2 lime (juiced)
- 1 tablespoon chia seeds
- 1 cup coconut water
- Ice cubes (optional)

Instructions:

- Blend the mango, basil leaves, lime juice, chia seeds, and coconut water until smooth.
- Adjust thickness with additional coconut water.
- Pour into a glass and enjoy the tropical mango-basil refresher!

Benefits:

Mango provides a sweet and tropical base, while basil adds a unique twist, offering antioxidants and anti-inflammatory benefits.

29. Raspberry Almond Spinach Smoothie

Ingredients:

- 1 cup raspberries
- 1/2 cup spinach leaves
- 1/2 cup almond milk
- 1 tablespoon almond flour
- 1 tablespoon honey
- Ice cubes (optional)

Instructions:

- Blend the raspberries, spinach, almond milk, almond flour, and honey until smooth.
- Adjust thickness with additional almond milk.
- Pour into a glass and enjoy the delightful raspberry-almond-spinach combination!

Benefits:

This smoothie combines the antioxidant power of raspberries with the nutrient-rich goodness of spinach and almonds.

30. Cucumber Kiwi Quencher

Ingredients:

- 1/2 cucumber (peeled and sliced)
- 2 kiwis (peeled and sliced)
- 1/2 lime (juiced)
- 1 tablespoon chia seeds
- 1 cup coconut water
- Ice cubes (optional)

Instructions:

- Blend the cucumber, kiwis, lime juice, chia seeds, and coconut water until smooth.
- Adjust thickness with additional coconut water.
- Pour into a glass and relish the hydrating cucumber-kiwi quencher!

Benefits:

Cucumber adds a refreshing element, while kiwi provides vitamin C and chia seeds contribute omega-3 fatty acids for added health benefits.

31. Cranberry Citrus Splash

Ingredients:

- 1/2 cup cranberries (fresh or frozen)

- 1/2 orange (peeled and segmented)

- 1/2 cup Greek yogurt

- 1 tablespoon honey

- 1 cup water or coconut water

- Ice cubes (optional)

Instructions:

- Blend the cranberries, orange segments, Greek yogurt, honey, and water or coconut water until smooth.

- Adjust thickness with additional liquid.

- Pour into a glass and enjoy the tart and refreshing cranberry citrus splash!

Benefits:

Cranberries provide a burst of antioxidants, while the citrus elements contribute vitamin C and immune-boosting properties.

32. Papaya Passion Fusion

Ingredients:

- 1 cup papaya chunks

- 1/2 banana

- 1/2 cup coconut milk

- 1 tablespoon chia seeds

- 1 tablespoon honey

- Ice cubes (optional)

Instructions:

- Blend the papaya, banana, coconut milk, chia seeds, and honey until smooth.
- Adjust thickness with additional coconut milk.
- Pour into a glass and relish the tropical and passion-filled papaya fusion!

Benefits:

Papaya offers digestive enzymes and antioxidants, while coconut milk adds creaminess and healthy fats to the smoothie.

33. Blackberry Basil Bliss

Ingredients:

- 1 cup blackberries
- 1/4 cup fresh basil leaves
- 1/2 cup plain yogurt
- 1 tablespoon almond butter
- 1 cup almond milk
- Ice cubes (optional)

Instructions:

- Blend the blackberries, basil leaves, yogurt, almond butter, and almond milk until smooth.

- Adjust thickness with additional almond milk.
- Pour into a glass and enjoy the unique and refreshing blackberry-basil bliss!

Benefits:

Blackberries provide antioxidants, while basil adds a fresh and aromatic twist, contributing potential anti-inflammatory benefits.

34. Mango Pineapple Turmeric Twist

Ingredients:

- 1 cup mango chunks
- 1/2 cup pineapple chunks
- 1/2 teaspoon turmeric powder
- 1 tablespoon chia seeds
- 1 cup coconut water
- Ice cubes (optional)

Instructions:

- Blend the mango, pineapple, turmeric powder, chia seeds, and coconut water until smooth.
- Adjust thickness with additional coconut water.
- Pour into a glass and savor the tropical and anti-inflammatory turmeric twist!

Benefits:

Mango and pineapple bring tropical sweetness, while turmeric adds anti-inflammatory properties to this vibrant smoothie.

35. Raspberry Lemonade Cooler

Ingredients:

- 1 cup raspberries
- 1/2 lemon (juiced)
- 1/2 cup Greek yogurt
- 1 tablespoon honey
- 1 cup water or coconut water
- Ice cubes (optional)

Instructions:

- Blend the raspberries, lemon juice, Greek yogurt, honey, and water or coconut water until smooth.
- Adjust thickness with additional liquid.
- Pour into a glass and enjoy the tart and revitalizing raspberry lemonade cooler!

Benefits:

Raspberries provide antioxidants, while the lemon adds a zesty kick, creating a refreshing and hydrating beverage.

36. Tropical Turmeric Dream

Ingredients:

- 1 cup pineapple chunks
- 1/2 teaspoon turmeric powder
- 1/2 cup coconut milk
- 1/2 banana
- 1 tablespoon chia seeds
- Ice cubes (optional)

Instructions:

- Blend pineapple, turmeric, coconut milk, banana, and chia seeds until smooth.
- Adjust thickness with additional coconut milk.
- Pour into a glass and indulge in the tropical turmeric dream!

Benefits:

Turmeric brings anti-inflammatory properties, while pineapple and coconut milk contribute a tropical twist and healthy fats.

37. Blueberry Lavender Serenity

Ingredients:

- 1 cup blueberries
- 1/2 teaspoon dried lavender (culinary-grade)

- 1/2 cup plain yogurt

- 1 tablespoon almond butter

- 1 cup almond milk

- Ice cubes (optional)

Instructions:

Blend blueberries, dried lavender, yogurt, almond butter, and almond milk until smooth.

Adjust thickness with additional almond milk.

Pour into a glass and experience the calming and flavorful blueberry lavender serenity!

Benefits:

Blueberries provide antioxidants, while lavender adds a unique and soothing element to this smoothie.

38. Green Tea Berry Infusion

Ingredients:

- 1/2 cup mixed berries (strawberries, blueberries, raspberries)

- 1/2 cup brewed green tea (cooled)

- 1/2 banana

- 1 tablespoon honey

- 1 cup coconut water

- Ice cubes (optional)

Instructions:

- Blend mixed berries, green tea, banana, honey, and coconut water until smooth.
- Adjust thickness with additional coconut water.
- Pour into a glass and enjoy the antioxidant-rich green tea berry infusion!

Benefits:

Green tea provides antioxidants, and combined with berries, it offers a refreshing and healthful beverage.

39. Peach Ginger Zing

Ingredients:

- 1 cup peach slices (fresh or frozen)
- 1/2 teaspoon ginger (grated)
- 1/2 cup plain yogurt
- 1 tablespoon honey
- 1 cup almond milk
- Ice cubes (optional)

Instructions:

- Blend peaches, ginger, yogurt, honey, and almond milk until smooth.

- Adjust thickness with additional almond milk.

- Pour into a glass and savor the zesty peach ginger zing!

Benefits:

Ginger brings anti-inflammatory properties, while peaches contribute a sweet and juicy flavor.

40. Berry Spinach Protein Power

Ingredients:

- 1 cup mixed berries (strawberries, blueberries)
- 1/2 cup spinach leaves
- 1/2 cup Greek yogurt
- 1 scoop protein powder (vanilla or berry flavor)
- 1 cup water or coconut water
- Ice cubes (optional)

Instructions:

Blend mixed berries, spinach, Greek yogurt, protein powder, and water or coconut water until smooth.

Adjust thickness with additional liquid.

Pour into a glass and enjoy the protein-packed berry spinach power!

Benefits:

This smoothie combines the goodness of berries with spinach and protein powder, providing a nutrient-rich and satisfying option.

CONCLUSION

incorporating nutrient-rich smoothies into the diet can be a flavorful and practical approach for individuals managing Sjögren's Syndrome. These recipes offer a diverse range of flavors and nutritional benefits, aiming to address specific concerns associated with this autoimmune condition.

From hydrating tropical blends to antioxidant-packed berry concoctions, each smoothie is carefully crafted to provide essential nutrients that may help alleviate symptoms and support overall well-being.

While smoothies can be a delicious addition to the daily routine, it's essential to recognize that they should complement, not replace, a well-balanced and varied diet. Individual nutritional needs may vary, and consulting with healthcare professionals, including registered dietitians, can help tailor dietary choices to specific requirements and preferences.

Moreover, maintaining a healthy lifestyle, staying well-hydrated, and prioritizing nutrient-dense foods are crucial aspects of managing Sjögren's Syndrome. Smoothies, enriched with key nutrients and hydration, can play a supportive role in enhancing the quality of life for individuals with this condition.